C.L.A.

The Essential Nutrient for Cutting Cancer Risk, Reducing Body Fat, and Providing Antioxidant Properties

LANE WILLIAMS

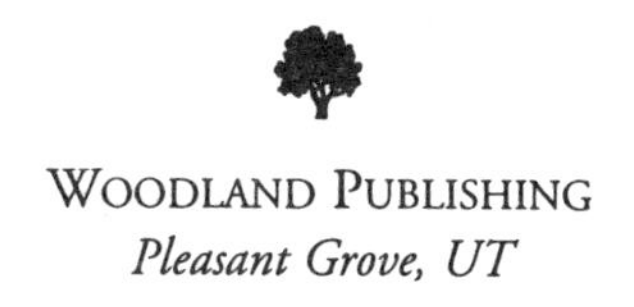

WOODLAND PUBLISHING
Pleasant Grove, UT

Woodland Publishing, Inc.
P.O. Box 160
Pleasant Grove, UT
84062

The information in this book is for educational purposes only and is not recommended as a means of diagnosing or treating an illness. All matters concerning physical and mental health should be supervised by a health practitioner knowledgeable in treating that particular condition. Neither the publisher nor author directly or indirectly dispense medical advice, nor do they prescribe any remedies or assume any responsibility for those who choose to treat themselves.

Table of Contents

Introduction

Next time someone you know puts a burger on a charcoal grill, notice how the fat drops, sizzling, onto the briquettes beneath As the drippings burn, the chemical content changes. This really is what burning is, a chemical change from a complex form of the substance to a more simple form. As it changes, many chemicals emerge—some harmless, others less so.

One of those chemicals, benzopyrene, can cause mutation of bacteria in the test tube, and that led some scientists to believe it might cause cancer.[1] Benzopyrene becomes part of the smoke that rises from the charcoal to settle back on the surface of a cooking burger. This was known as far back as the 1970s, and, for those interested in good health, it became another reason to cut meats from the diet and replace them with healthy grains and vegetable products.

Many left it at that. Thankfully, scientists began digging more deeply into this phenomenon, measuring other chemicals and other methods of cooking. One such scientist was Michael Pariza. In 1978, Pariza studied heterocyclic amines to see if they were "mutagenic," that is, if they would cause bacteria to mutate in the test tube. He found that burgers can be quite safely cooked with care.[2]

But what changed the direction of his research was an entirely original discovery, separate from what his paper set out to find. This discovery has shaped his career since and may well, in the years to come, help thousands, indeed millions, of people improve their health. What he discovered was that something in hamburger has a "mutagenic inhibitory" effect. That is, something in meat seemed to counteract the bad effects of these mutagens, indeed was an anti-mutagen.

In his research, Pariza used a popular scientific test called the Ames Test, named for a scientist at the University of California at Berkeley. This test is still used today for its simplicity by numerous scientists. The test requires enzymes form rat livers stimulated with certain chemicals. Scientists put these enzymes and the possible mutagen onto bacteria. They observe the bacteria in a microscope to see if they have mutated.

Pariza changed the experiment slightly. Instead of stimulating rat livers, he used enzymes from normal rat livers. The results showed this anti-mutagenic effect, but just what substance caused it was still a question. For nearly another decade, Pariza and others tried to isolate this substance. Finally, they managed to do so in 1987.[3] Call it a previously undiscovered nutrient, one, by the best research now available, that seems essentially vital for optimal health. The substance is CLA—conjugated linoleic acid. Laboratory studies using animals show:

- CLA has powerful anti-cancer potential.
- It seems to help keep arteries from getting clogged as easily.
- It helps a body deal with the cascade of effects that occurs when an infection sets in, helping animals, and potentially humans.
- It can help cut body fat while building lean muscle tissue, and that means animals are healthier and, perhaps, lose weight.

• Though this question is debated, many researchers believe it is a powerful antioxidant as well.

Significantly, because of modern agricultural techniques, the amount of CLA in our diets today is much lower than it used to be, and that may, at least in part, explain America's growing girth.

An Essential Fatty Acid

When most people think of fat, they think of the white gooey stuff that deposits around the waist or around the thighs. In many ways, it can be tempting to spell it "fatt"—making it an unspeakable, four-letter word.

But at the level of the cell, at the level of molecules, fat means something more complicated. First of all, fat is one method the body uses to store energy for long periods. When we eat, we must either immediately burn the fuel as energy, or store it as fat or as protein for muscle. Fat, therefore, is one way our body tries to make something useful from food. Furthermore, fat serves a vital function in each cell. The membranes of our cells are all made of fat—a collection of fatty acids really. Every cellular function must pass through this barrier. Hormones act on fat, energy passes through fat, life proceeds because of fat.

Fat, then, is not a dirty word. It is vital. Scientists have identified more than 100 fatty acids, and many more fatty acids could theoretically exist.[4] The body produces all the fatty acids it needs except three—linoleic acid, arachadonic acid and linolinic acid. Much the way certain vitamins like vitamin C are essential to good health and are not produced naturally, these acids are essential, hence their name—essential fatty acids. The body can produce linolinic acid and arachadonic acid from linoleic acid, so in some senses, the only vital fatty acid is linoleic acid.

Linoleic acid sits like a highway of some 58 atoms of carbon, oxygen and hydrogen.[5] The carbon is the center line with the hydrogen and oxygen being the cars traveling along the way. (Thousands of chemicals contain these three elements in nature. It is the order of these cars, and the varied shapes of the highway, that lead to many different kinds of chemicals.)

The highway of linoleic acid sits curved like a mountain switchback. Conjugated linoleic acid is basically a straighter version of linoleic acid. Scientists have studied CLA at least since the 1930s.[6] These studies show that bacteria in the stomach convert linoleic acid into CLA.[7]

CLA occurs naturally in many foods including some vegetable oils, which are the best sources for linoleic acid, but the best source of CLA is in beef, veal and certain dairy products.[8] Dr. Mark Cook, who began working with Pariza around1990, said the reason that sheep and cows and other similar animals provide higher sources of CLA is because these animals are ruminants—they have multiple stomachs for bacteria to convert linoleic acid in, instead of one, as in humans.[9]

The chemistry of CLA really isn't that significant to any but a researcher, but, in essence, a double bond of two of the carbon atoms switches position from its position in linoleic acid.[10] Instead of having two atoms between a pair of double chemical bonds, as in linoleic acid, there is only one atom in between. This is why chemists named it conjugated linoleic acid. This chemical chain can exist in several forms with the double bonds at positions 9 and 11, positions 11 and 13 or at positions 10 and 12.[11] Hence, there are several forms of CLA.

Which ones are most effective in providing nutrition, or if they are equally effective, is still a question somewhat unresolved, although it is unlikely that it is the 11,13 version.[12]

What has been resolved is that CLA is one of the most important, and most exciting nutrients isolated in recent years. And there's good reason to look at supplementing it into your diet. Why? Because we may not be getting as much of it as we once did, particularly in the United States.[13]

Cows and other animals have traditionally eaten fresh grasses as a way of getting nutrition, but agricultural development makes it more efficient and cost-effective to provide cattle feed grains and other means of nutrition, instead of natural grasses. That seems to mean that the cows today provide much less CLA in their beef than those of only a generation ago. One study out of Australia showed that cattle in that South Pacific nation had more than twice the amount of CLA than American cows. The reason may well be differences in feeding patterns.

As evidence for this, have you ever wondered why it is that Americans, despite eating less fat and meat than a generation ago, end up being more fat than their predecessors? Indeed, America's obesity rate is up substantially over the last 15 years.[14] Declining amounts of CLA may explain this disturbing trend. But more on that later.

CLA and Cancer

Because of Pariza's 1979 research, some of the earliest studies done on CLA were to see if it could block the development of cancer. Dr. Pariza and his colleagues at the University of Wisconsin/Madison's Food Research Institute in Madison took extracts from beef that they knew had "mutagen modulators" (this was before they isolated CLA.).[15] They took two groups of mice, to one they applied this extract on their skin. On the other group, they did not apply the extract on the skin. Then, on both sets, researchers put a cancer-causing substance called dimethylbenaanthracene—DMBA for short—and applied it to the skin.

Sixteen weeks later, doctors counted the mice that had tumors and how many tumors each of those mice had. The number of mice with tumors was 20 percent lower when given the beef extract, and, significantly, the numbers of tumors on those mice that did develop cancer was half what it was on the untreated mice. This meant that this extract could, perhaps, prevent some cancers in mice and, slow tumors after they develop. (Today, Pariza writes that CLA inhibits cancer development at various stages, from initiation to metastasis.)[16] After isolating CLA by itself, Pariza and others found that CLA also cut the incidence of skin tumors.[17]

Scientist Clement Ip at the Roswell Park Cancer Institute in Buffalo did a similar study using DMBA with rats, this time feeding different amounts of CLA into the diet and over a longer period of time. He and his team measured how many breast tumors these rats developed. As might have been expected with the earlier work, 20 percent fewer animals developed the tumors—among those receiving the most CLA—than the rats that received none, and the total number of tumors that developed was 60 percent less. In general, the data showed that the more CLA, the greater the protective effect.[18]

This is significant in the human world because many researchers see a link between a woman's consumption of fat and her risk of getting breast cancer, and CLA could help modulate that. Any research to lower a woman's chance of contracting breast cancer is useful. Today in the United States, as many as one in eight will contract the dread disease.[19]

In 1990, Dr. Pariza and his colleagues also found a lower incidence of cancers in parts of the stomach.[20] Rats were given something called 2-amino-3-methylimidazo (4,5-f]quinoline, which can give them colon cancer. Again, the total number of aberrant growths was lower for those given CLA compared with those given safflower oil, which is rich in essential oils but not so high in CLA.[21]

Does this mean that CLA will prevent cancer in humans? Perhaps. You might even say probably—in some circumstances Still, science can be imprecise in predicting cancers from animal models to humans, and scientific tests must be controlled in ways that don't mimic the complexities and confounding factors of daily life. Few of us, for example, will be exposed daily to DMBA. Therefore, all the science says for certain is that CLA seems to hinder the development of cancer in these animals when the cancer is caused by one particular substance. That's a little way, at least, from saying it prevents cancers in humans.

However, the animal models are encouraging, and often meet mathematical tests to be "statistically significant." In fact, scientists have taken to saying CLA has an anti-carcinogenic effect without hedging. Ip himself says, "CLA is more powerful than any other fatty acid in modulating tumor development."[22] Indeed, so excited have many scientists become that some say one day governments may want to fortify our foods with CLA much the way we fortify our morning bran flakes with vitamin C.[23] Furthermore, since at least several ways of giving different species of animals cancer have been studied, and in all of the tests, cancer was hindered, it gives better evidence to the notion that CLA hinders cancer in humans as well. Pariza wrote, "Few anticarcinogens, and certainly no other known fatty acids, are as effective as CLA in inhibiting carcinogenesis in these models."[24] This is clear language saying scientist believe this to be a powerful nutrient in the war against cancer. However, until human research is completed, and human research is underway, the positive effects of CLA on humans as a possible preventative of cancer best be considered preliminary.

Another important point about this is: Since the breakdown and changing of fats and fatty acids like CLA occur in the liver, CLA may have unknown effects on this vital organ. One study showed that fats increase in the livers with the increase of CLA in the diet.[25] Could this lead to an increased risk of liver cancer? Scientists do not have a complete answer to that question either.[26] Pariza says, however, that such problems of fat accumulation do not occur in higher mammals, and is something specific to mice and some rats.[27]

How Does CLA Work?

How could CLA hinder the growth and development of certain cancers in animals? Scientists have developed some intriguing possibilities, and many of them are related to the theory of antioxidants.

WHAT IS AN ANTIOXIDANT?

Well, one of the ironies of life is that oxygen, so essential to human life, also causes decay. Look at the parts of your car where paint may have pealed away, and you will notice rust, what scientists call oxidation. Molecules of oxygen combine with the iron or chromium on your car and change its chemical alignment to iron oxide or chromium oxide—rust.

In a very real sense, the same thing happens to you as you age. Inside your cells, thousands of chemical reactions take place each moment. These reactions break apart the long chains of carbon, oxygen and hydrogen that make up body tissues and combines them in new ways. Some of those combinations cause decay. One example is when a free radical—a single atom of roaming oxygen—attaches itself to something useful, rendering it useless or even dangerous. If a free radical were to change DNA, for example, that could mutate a cell.

This free radical process is one way this oxidation occurs, and antioxidants, often called free radical scavengers, attach themselves to the free radicals, blocking their damage. This can help improve life and help to cut the problems of oxidation. Indeed, many see antioxidants as a way of lessening the risks of cancer.

Many people know about important antioxidants, such as ascorbigen (vitamin C), selenium or alpha tocopherol (vitamin E), but nature provides numerous antioxidants. Many exciting ones are emerging, such as proanthocyanidins (often known as pycnogenol), quercetin (common in many fruits) and selenium (a mineral).

CLA may be another antioxidant emerging from the research. Dr. Pariza and others found in a 1991 experiment that in the test tube, CLA was effective in battling free radicals.[28] It helped prevent damage to the DNA inside the cells. Pariza says in another paper, "Our hypothesis is that the antioxidant activity of CLA may at least in part explain its anticarcinogenic effect."[29] That would mean that one way CLA prevents cancer is because it blocks these dangerous free radicals. (Other theories about how it fights cancer include breaking down the chemicals that cause cancer into others that don't .[30] All the theories may be true in specific situations, and none might.)

But like many other emerging, exciting areas of scientific inquiry, this idea that CLA is an antioxidant has doubters. Researchers J.J. van den Berg, N.E. Cook and D.L. Tribble wanted to see if CLA protected fatty membranes comprised of a substance called palmitoyl-2-linoleoyl phosphatidylcholine (PLPC) from the damage of biologic oxidation. In research published in 1995, they compared CLA's effect to the well-known antioxidant vitamin E. While vitamin E protected well, CLA did relatively little. They also found that CLA did not become a mineral chelator, an agent that helps natural minerals become available biologically. They bluntly said, "On the basis of our observations, a role for CLA as an antioxidant does not seem plausible."[31]

Another study in 1995, however, showed that CLA can break down into other substances, called feran derivatives, that do act as antioxidants.[32] As in all emerging sciences, debates ensue among honest, dedicated researchers. CLA may not, itself, be a antioxidant. Perhaps it acts as antioxidant in only certain situations. Perhaps things that come from CLA act like antioxidants. That is the state of the research today. (Indeed, Dr. Pariza says such debates are common in the field of antioxidants.[33])

What is important to remember is that in numerous animal models, CLA protected against the dangers of many different kinds of cancer in animals, and that, according to scientists, it is one of the most potent cancer-preventing substances of its kind known to science. Whether the cause of this effect was because of CLA or because of some other reason really isn't that important.

Another thing to remember is that CLA is not a cancer drug. It is something that would be useful in addition to other cancer treatments. It is something to consider to lower your risks and, perhaps, lessen the effects of treatment. It should not be considered a treatment option on its own.

CLA and Atherosclerosis

CLA may well have benefits in the battle against heart disease as well. The leading cause of death in the United States is heart disease or related diseases of the circulatory system. Indeed, U.S. statistics show that about half the people in the United States die that way.

In 1989, for example, some 2 million Americans died, and about 950,000 of those died as a direct or indirect result of heart disease. That's far more than the total number of deaths from AIDS, shootings, bombings and accidents combined.[34] For perspective, let's discuss what happens when a newsworthy accident occurs—let's say an airline crash that kills 200 people. Statistically speaking, five times that many people will die the same day of heart disease, as many as two each minute.

Thankfully, doctors have made great progress in battling these conditions, and researchers have discovered that a healthy lifestyle can help the heart. Indeed, as almost everyone knows, balanced nutrition, lower stress and plenty of exercise can lead a person to be more healthy and to run a lower risk of heart attack and other heart conditions.

Evidently, at least in animals, CLA seems to possess the ability to cut risks as well. Dr. Pariza and two colleagues, Kisun Lee and David Kritchevsky, studied a group of 12 rabbits that were fed a diet high in fat and cholesterol. They gave six of them CLA. In the academic journal *Atherosclerosis,* they reported that two dangerous compounds, LDL cholesterol and triglycerides, were "markedly lower" in the six that had diets supplemented with CLA.

When the scientists looked at the aortas—the largest artery leading from the heart—of these animals, they also found a lot less blockage than in those that didn't have CLA. This is how they summarized their results: "CLA appears to be hypocholesterolemic and anti-atherogenic."[35] This is pretty bold stuff for cautious scientists. Though the words are complex, the statement is clear: CLA seems to cut cholesterol and makes it so veins won't clog as easily.

This finding was surprising to Dr. Pariza. Science shows that straightened fatty acids (trans-fatty acids) of which CLA is one, usually tend to increase the risk of heart disease. Pariza said it only made sense to test CLA with this kind of science. Indeed, the best he would hope for would be no effect.[36] In 1996, another group studied atherosclerosis and hamsters supplementing diets with CLA. CLA didn't cut the amount of cholesterol in the blood within three months, but it did cut the amount of fatty build-up in the aorta of the hamsters.[37]

The bottom line on heart disease and CLA? Because two different types of animals show less clogging of the arteries, it seems clear that a good chance exists for the same thing to happen in humans. Of course, as with the cancer research, solid studies in humans need to be conducted for researchers to say definitely that this can cut your risk of heart disease.

But until that day, the news is good: A nutritional regimen that includes solid antioxidants like vitamin C and vitamin A, that includes magnesium,[38] coenzyme Q10,[39] and that includes other important circulatory system-fortifiers would likely benefit from CLA. Couple that nutrition with a healthful lifestyle, and your chances of living longer and living better will likely increase.

CLA and the Catabolic Cascade

Next fall, when you or a friend goes to the doctor to get a flu shot, notice how a low-grade fever starts. Notice how rundown you or your friend begin to feel for a day or so after the shot. It is as if you are dealing with a small portion of the disease.

In some respects you are, but, in reality, the icky, yucky feelings we associate with sickness come from our body's own response to an invasion. When the immune system goes on the offensive, it puts out hormones called cytokines. Those cytokines cause fever and pain.

Doctors call this process the catabolic cascade. It is our body that produces it. An extreme example might have been when

Jim Henson, the wonderful creator of Kermit the Frog, got an extreme bacterial infection. He died within about 12 hours. Although the bacteria caused some severe reactions, it was his body's intense catabolic response that may have been the direct cause of death.

Cytokines are involved in more than just stimulating the immune system, they are involved in how the body accumulates fat, in how veins accumulate deposits and in how our body during disease can sometimes cause dangerous, rapid weight loss. CLA changes how cytokines work, but how it does it is not certain.

Here's an example of why this is important: When young animals get sick, their immune systems kick into action. Besides contracting a fever, the animals' growth slows. Furthermore, weight and muscle mass can be lost, not just because of loss of appetite, but because of degradation of muscle tissue. For a poultry farmer, this can be significant. In organized farms, bacteria can abound and young chicks often face sickness. Because their immune systems are firing, the cytokines can stunt growth and, accordingly, stunt the farmer's profits.

Dr. Mark Cook was working on this dilemma in 1990 and jogging at the campus of the University of Wisconsin-Madison. During one of his regular exercise sessions, he began chatting with Dr. Pariza. As researchers do, they began talking about their work. They decided to collaborate, seeing if CLA had an effect on this problem.

In 1993, the scientists at the University of Wisconsin--Madison injected rat pups with endotoxin, the substances bacteria produce to do their damage.[40] This injection activated their immune systems. They also did the same thing in two studies using chicks. In all three studies, the weight-loss was about half what it was during the other studies.

In a study published in 1994, researchers also injected endotoxin into mice. To some, they gave CLA, to others they didn't After three days, the scientists weighed the mice and discovered that those who also received CLA in their diets lost much less weight. Indeed, after three days they weighed as much as the control group, which received no endotoxin at all. The CLA-fed group also had a much better appetite than those that received no CLA with endotoxin. They also had a higher muscle mass.[41]

Let's repeat that. CLA gives a higher muscle mass in rats. Stop and think about the implications. Other studies have shown, and, we will get to them, that CLA also cuts the amount of food converted to fat. In an era of increasing battles with the bulge, CLA seems to show great promise. (That weight gain seems to be involved somehow with the immune system and cytokines indicates that working with cytokines may be how CLA affects body fat accumulation.)

Yes, CLA can help cut the effects of immune stimulation, but does it do that at the expense of making our immune systems less effective? Does CLA affect how the body battles disease? Not from any evidence in any study. The 1993 studies measured several immune functions, and, if anything, the immune system worked better.[42]

Again, these are animal studies, not necessarily involved with how humans work. However, these studies involve more than one kind of animal, making it, again, more likely to be useful in humans.

Let's speculate for a minute. When CLA cuts the catabolic cascade, doesn't it make sense that the body would feel better, if only because the appetite is better? When CLA cuts weight loss, couldn't that have immense benefits for patients suffering from long-term illnesses—including those illnesses that affect the immune system—who grow weak from a loss of muscle tone and from a loss of weight?

For the animal industry, of course, this nutrient clearly means better production methods and healthier animals. For those same animals, it seems possible to speculate that CLA may actually work as a growth factor for their young.[43] For humans, this nutrient could mean feeling better and feeling stronger while the body fights off disease.

At the beginning of this booklet, we learned that CLA may be one of the most important nutrients discovered in recent years. The support for that statement should be clear. CLA, if the human studies hold true, could cut your risk for cancer, could lower your risk of heart disease, could help you feel better when you are ill, and improve muscle tone while decreasing body fat.

This research has one other interesting side effect. Cook says that during much of the research, graduate students helping in the work would continually report that animals were eating less. Indeed, the animals ate up to 30 percent less while gaining weight or helping the immune system.

If all animals in the world were fed CLA, and it cut feed intake by 30 percent, this would have strong implications on world starvation and feed efficiency. Especially in a world where meat consumption may be growing. Cutting the amount of animal feed necessary to produce the same number of animals is vital. This, too, is a possible result of CLA.[44]

CLA and Body Fat

Of all the health concerns facing Americans today, few are as important and daunting as weight loss and body fat. In the 1980s, Americans gained an average of eight pounds each. That's on the order of 1 million tons of flab—2 billion total American pounds.[45] So large is the current girth that as many as two in three Americans could be termed overweight.[46] Being overweight and having excess fat increases the risk of heart disease, some forms of cancer and diabetes. That collection of health challenges would be difficult enough, but being overweight has many problems that accompany it, including battles with self-esteem.

Let's give a historical example of this story. The emotional power of being perceived as too fat is caught with pathos in the life of former U.S. President William Howard Taft. Taft, who is the only man to serve as both president and as chief justice of the Supreme Court, was noted for his honesty and his integrity. The nation mourned his death, but much of his internal story focused on his battle with weight.

One editorial cartoonist showed the island of Cuba tipping under his girth. Once, when he visited Japan, an entire village worked together to pull his rickshaw up a hill. When he married, his personal esteem showed when he told his wife that "I shall worry you so much with my appetite that you must gain strength to meet the trial."

Taft refused to be seen on a horse because of how awkward he looked. At one point, he lost 75 pounds, but, like so many others, ended up gaining that amount back , and more, during the next 10 years. He died of atherosclerosis, something associated with being overweight.[47] The tragedy of Taft is that, like so many suffering with weight trouble, he seemed to let it damage his self worth, when he was a great asset to his nation and to others.

History and culture put into us that being overweight means lacking in self-control and being a glutton, when in reality this isn't true. So many more factors are involved. Each person has a different metabolism. Certain nutrients can meet different needs, and a lack of those nutrients can lead to fat retention.

CLA may be one of those nutrients, one of those factors in our diets that can change our shapes and that have nothing to do with self-control, just nutritional luck and knowledge.

In a study of rats, 28 days after beginning the study, body fat in those that ate CLA was 58 percent less than in those who didn't consume any (10.13 percent body fat versus 4.34 percent body fat, a highly significant difference). Also, the percent of muscle was about one percent more in animals that ate CLA. The weights of both sets of animals were about the same.[48] (Muscle weighs more than fat. This can mean that you won't necessarily lose weight with CLA, but would gain muscle mass, which is tighter and more shapely.)

The research in this area is slightly newer, but it has been reproduced in studies on other animals.[49] That more than one kind of animal has shown that body fat is lower with supplements of CLA indicates that it will likely benefit humans as well.

In July 1997, preliminary results of one of the first human studies involving CLA showed promising, preliminary results. For three months in 1997, 20 volunteers participated in a study, daily consuming an amount of slightly more than one gram of CLA at breakfast lunch and dinner. Three months later, their weights and body-fat percents were measured. Half of the group took a placebo. The average weight of the 10 who took CLA dropped by about five pounds (not enough to be statistically significant), but the body fat percentage dropped by about 15 to 20 percent, or from 21.3 percent of average body fat to 17 percent of body fat. Meanwhile, the group taking a placebo had little or no effect on either.

Half of the people in the study were men and half were women. Two people in the study decided to drop out because they received unpleasant gastrointestinal upsets. One of those who dropped out was in the placebo group, the other in the group taking CLA.[63]

Nobody would suggest that CLA supplementation would be a pill freeing you to sit slug-like on the couch to watch

M*A*S*H* reruns. A healthy, weight-conscious lifestyle requires many factors including exercise. As far as science can tell, CLA may not be essential the way certain vitamins are. If you consume no vitamin C, you can expect to get scurvy and die. There are no known deficiency diseases associated with an absence of CLA.

Japanese consumers, for example, get very little CLA in their diets, but they also eat food very low in fat, and their lives are among the longest in the world.[50] So, the role of CLA supplementation in regulating weight is most useful for those with a typically high-fat Western diet. As the science grows, it seems clear that CLA will lead to better health and more hope for people struggling with body fat.

CLA and Cows

Nutritional developments like that of CLA couldn't come at a better time. America is a nation obsessed with weight, but successes in battling weight seem harder and harder to come by.

Is there a nutritional reason for this? Have we been barking up the wrong tree in recent years, starving ourselves for fear of gluttony rather than looking at broader nutritional reasons for fat accumulation? For example, Dr. Cook says that modern nutritional dogma is that fat is bad. "I'm not sure the dogma's right. We need to get down to very specific fatty acids."[51]

One of the most exciting developments coming from CLA research is that modern animal-raising techniques may be partially responsible for those of us who eat meat getting fat around the middle, even though our consumption of meat may have declined or, at least, stayed about the same in recent years. CLA has been declining in our diet. This one nutrient's lack may mean many of us are gaining fat, despite eating less overall fat.[52]

This desire to simply eliminate fats without looking at the broader nutritional picture has its roots deep in our culture. The desire to starve ourselves to lose weight goes back centuries. We have often thought weight gain came solely from lacking self-control when, often, nothing could be further from the truth.

Take for example the experiences of conscientious objectors during World War II. These men who chose, for religious reasons, not to fight in the war, contributed in other ways. One group at the University of Minnesota underwent forced starvation to help scientists learn ways to help concentration camp victims recover after liberation.

Science learned many useful things, but one thing stands out. The objectors grew more hungry as they recovered and ended up weighing five percent more after they recovered than before the experiment began. (The same can be said for refugees and concentration camp victims, who also weighed more, on average after their ordeals than before.)[53]

This idea of dieting being the full answer to weight loss still persists, often tragically. Many have died of anorexia, obsessed with self-image. Others have died directly from ill-conceived meal replacement programs.[54] In the 1980s, Americans spent $15 billion on diet soft drinks alone,[55] but consumers weighed more on average when the decade was over than when it began.

You'd think all of this energy and dieting spent on the effort would have helped people lose weight. (Thankfully, many people have succeeded in losing weight and keeping it off. According to Dr. Pariza, this may well be the most significant part of CLA, not so much in losing the weight, but in helping people keep it off.[56])

To drive the point home further, consider your parents. They ate a diet that was likely higher in fat than yours. They never saw "lite" versions of snacks in the store. Yet they, in general, weighed less than we do. Why? Surely exercise may have had something to do with it, but, no one has the complete answer. It seems likely that nutrition too played a role. CLA itself may hold part of the reason. As we have seen, CLA nutrition means less fat and more protein in our bodies.

Recent research is showing that the amount of CLA in cows has dropped substantially since the times of our parents. In 1963, scientists found that CLA was as much as 2.81 percent of milkfat. The amount of CLA in the milk products varied with the seasons. At some times during the year, cows ate grass. At other times, they ate feed. However, in 1992, Pariza and his colleagues did a large food survey and found that this variation in CLA is no longer occurring. Furthermore, the amount of CLA in dairy products rarely gets above 1 percent of the milkfat.[57]

In another research paper in 1994, scientists noticed that Australian cows have as much as three or four time the amount of CLA in the meat from similar American animals. Why? These differences probably "reflect different feeding conditions."[58] Today, farmers use more efficient feeding methods that rely less heavily on natural grasses. This means less CLA in the meat we eat, and less CLA can mean a higher percentage of fat on our bodies. Consider too that skim milk contains virtually no CLA with its no fat content. This lack of CLA may actually hinder some people's efforts to lose weight.

The lesson here seems to be that gluttony guilt would be better focused on balanced living. Healthy lifestyles coupled with the right supplementation can make a difference. CLA, though no magic bullet, adds to this lifestyle and could be the key that finally opens many weight (and fat) management doors. It could help many people keep the weight off.

How Much CLA is the Right Amount?

That is one question for researchers to answer with detailed human studies, but if you extrapolate from university studies on animals, it could be between two and six grams a day. (Some animal studies were actually at higher levels, to one half of one percent in weight of a day's calories.)

Some other things to consider:

- Watch the labels closely on supplements advertising that they contain CLA. CLA is present in many foods, and some marketers have capitalized on CLA science by simply putting vegetable oil in their supplements. Only a few supplements provide high levels of CLA. Select only those products that do.[59]
- Aside from questions about liver cancer, no adverse side effects have been reported in the scientific literature concerning CLA. CLA can probably be taken safely with other nutritional supplements, but fat-absorbing supplements like chitosan may actually absorb CLA, so it is useful to avoid taking the two products at the same time. Consider taking CLA in the morning and chitosan after high-fat meals.
- CLA is not like aspirin, in that it takes a few weeks, perhaps three, for its effects to be noticeable.[60]
- To get enough CLA from burgers, you would probably have to eat about two pounds a day, not something recommended given beef's high fat content.
- In general, plants have virtually no CLA.
- Two of the best natural sources of CLA are beef and veal.
- An interesting side of the research is now emerging. According to Cook, in animal studies trying to study the amount of fat and muscle in an animal, they noticed consistently, that overall weight was up. Most recently, as yet unpub-

lished results show that bone mass is increased in pigs who take CLA. This has huge implications for research into osteoporosis, and research into this field is underway.[61]

Some Final Thoughts

One of the important proofs of the belief Pariza and Cook have in this supplement is to learn that they both take it themselves. Cook says it is the only supplement he takes, and he believes he will take it the rest of his life. He was naturally thin because of intense exercise, but he believes that it has helped him to keep inches off during long weeks of travel.

Pariza, for his part, has lost three inches from his waist during the last year, as well as about seven pounds. He said he has less of an appetite. He says he feels warmer, probably an effect of a faster metabolism. He warns that this is not a quick fix. When he first started taking this supplement, he found virtually no results. He was disappointed. But the results have come.[62]

Another significant thing to remember is that, today, scores of scientists around the country are now studying this nutrient. The results will pile in human studies and in other long-term clinical trials. These will give broad indications of the use of this natural, previously unrecognized nutrient.

Why would CLA be involved in so many functions? If human studies hold true, and the expectation is that they will, you might consider this the next aspirin or the next vitamin C. Vital, remarkable nutrients seem to work on a basic level and impact a variety of systems. This is the case with CLA. What a remarkable piece of science that emerged from a charcoal grill.

So, the next time charcoal briquettes sizzle with the drippings of a nice burger, remember how science has found that life, with its remarkable chemistry, finds a way to survive and thrive. No better example exists than that beef cooking on the grill. Sizzling steak covers itself with dangerous chemicals that can cause cancer. Many people feared that fact for years, and science studied those dangers earnestly. How encouraging that nature thankfully also provided other chemicals that counteract, partially at least, the effects of these dangers.

CLA, just another highway of chemicals, is a quiet blessing, wiping out carcinogens, blocking dangerous fat, and striving to keep our veins clear. And it was there all along, doing its job, just waiting to be studied and understood.

Now that nearly two decades of research are beginning to show how this substance can benefit our lives, a celebration of nature's bounty seems to be in order. Let's light up the old grill. Shall we make it steaks or burgers this time?

REFERENCES

1. Interview with Dr. Michael Pariza, July 3, 1997.
2. "Effects of Temperature and Time on Mutagen Formation in Pan-Fried Hamburger," by M. Pariza, Samy Ashoor, Fun Chu and Daryl Lund, March 10, 1979, Cancer Letters, 7 (1979) 63-69.
3. "Anticarcinogens from fried ground beef: heat-altered derivatives of linoleic acid," Y.L Ha, N.K. Grimm and M.W. Pariza, August 25, 1987. IRL Press limited, Oxford, England.
4. Interview with Dr. Mark Cook, July 3, 1997.
5. "Conjugated Linoleic Acid in Cancer Prevention Research: A Report of Current Status and Issues," A special report prepared for the National Live Stock and Meat Board, Ip, Clement, Ph.D., May 1994. See also "Conjugated linoleic acid, a newly recognised nutrient" in the June 17, 1997, issue of *Chemistry and Industry* by M. Pariza, pp. 464-466.
6. Op.Cit. Pariza, *Chemistry and Industry.*
7. Op. Cit. Ip, National Live Stock and Meat Board. See also, "Conjugated Linoleic Acid (9,11 and 10,12-Octadecadienoic Acid) is Produced in Conventional by Not Germ-Free Rats Fed Linleic Acid," Sou F. Chin, Et.

Al, Dec. 16, 1993, *Journal of Nutrition* 124: 694-701 1994.
8. Ibid.
9. Interview with Cook.
10. Op. Cit. Ip, National Live Stock and Meat Board.
11. Ibid.
12. Op. Cit., interview with Pariza., and "Anticarcinogens from fried ground beef: heat-altered derivatives of linoleic acid," Y.L. Ha, N.K. Grimm and M.W. Pariza, Aug. 25, 1987, IRL Press Limited, Oxford England.
13. "Conjugated linoleic acid: An anticarcinogenic fatty acid present in mile fat," by Peter Parodi, *Australian Journal of Dairy Technology.* Nov. 1994, 49 p. 93-94.
14. *The Washington Post* "Now We're a Nation of Lite Heavyweights," Sept. 1, 1994, Sec. B. P. 10.
15. "A beef-derived mutagenesis modulator inhibits initiation of mouse epidermal tumors by 7, 12 dimethylbens[a]anthracene," by M. Pariza and W. Hargraves, Jan. 2, 1985, *Carcinogenesis,* vol 6., no. 4 pp. 591-593, 1985, IRL Press, Limited, Oxford, England.
16. Op. Cit. Pariza, *Chemistry and Industry.*
17. "Anticarcinogens from fried ground beef: heat-altered derivatives of linoleic acid," Y.L. Ha, N.K. Grimm and M.W. Pariza, Aug. 25, 1987, IRL Press Limited, Oxford England.
18. "Mammary Cancer Prevention by Conjugated Dienoic Derivative of Linoleic Acid," Clement Ip, Sou Fe Chin, Joseph Scimeca and Michael Pariza, Cancer Research, 51, 6118-6124, Nov. 15, 1991.
19. "Refiguring the Odds: What's a woman's real chance of suffering breast cancer?" Facklemann, K.A., *Science News* 144 (1993) 76-77.
20. "Inhibition of benzo(a)pyrene-induced mouse forestomach neoplasia by conjugated dienoic derivatives of linoleic acid." Ha, Y.L, Storkson, J., Pariza, M.W. *Cancer Research* 50: 1097-1101; 1990.
21. "Protection of Conjugated linoleic acid against 2-amino-3-methylimidazo [4,5-f]quinoline-induced colon carcinogenesis in the f344 rat: a study of inhibitory mechanisims," Liew, C.; Schut, H.A.J., chin, S.F., Pariza, M.W., and Dashwood, R.H. (1995), *Carcinogenesis* 16, 3037-3044.
22. Op. Cit., Ip, Cancer Research, 1991.
23. "Potential of Food Modification in Cancer Prevention," Ip, C.; Lisk, Donald J. and J. Scimeca, *Cancer Research,* 54, 1957-1959, April 1, 1994.
24. "Conjugated Linoleic Acid (CLA), A Newly Recognized Anitcarcinogenic Nutrient," unpublished paper by Michael Pariza.
25. "Effects of conjugated dienoic linoleic acid on lipid metabolism in mouse liver," Belury, M.A. and Vanden Heuvel, J.P. (1996), Proc. Am.

Assoc. *Cancer Res.* 37: 1918.
26. "Protection Against Cancer and Heart Disease by Dietary Fatty Acid, Conjugated Linoleic Acid: Potential Mechanisms of Action," Belury, M.A.; Vanden Heuvel, J.P; Submitted to *Nutrition and Disease Update Journal,* Sept. 28, 1996.
27. Interveiw with Pariza.
28. Op. Cit., Pariza, *Cancer Research,* 1990.
29. "Fatty Acids that Inhibit Cancer," unpublished paper by M. Pariza.
30. Op. Cit. Liew.
31. "Reinvestigation of the antioxidant properties of conjugated linoleic acid," van den Berg J.J.; Cook, N.E.; Tribble D.L.; *Lipids,* 73, 1995, Jul 30 (7), 595-598.
32. "Furan Fatty acids detrmined as oxidation products of conjugated octadecadienoic acid," Yurawecz, M.P., Hood, J.K., Mossoba, MM., Roach, J.A.G., and Ku, Y. *Lipids* 30, 595-598.
33. Interview with Pariza.
34. "Vital Statistics of the United States" from the Centers for Disease Control for 1989.
35. "Conjugated linoleic acid and atherosclerosis in rabbits." Lee, K.N., Kritchevsky, D. And Pariza, M.W.; *Atherosclerosis* 108, 19-25.
36. Interview with Pariza.
37. "Dietary conjugated linoleic acid reduces aortic fatty streak formation greater than linoleic acid in hypercholesterolemic hamsters," Nicolosi, R.J., and Laitinen, L. (1996), FASEB J. 10 A477.
38. "Ionic Basis of Hypertension, Insulin in Resistance, Vascular Disease and Related Disorders. The Mechanism of 'Syndrome X", Resnick, LM, *American Journal of Hypertension.* 1993 (4Suppl) 123S-134S.
39. "Protection by coenzyme Q10 from myocardial reperfusion injury during coronary artery bypass grafting," Chello-M, et. Al, Ann-Thorac. *Surg.,* 1994, Nov; 58(5): 1427-32.
40. "Immune Modulation by Altered Nutrient Metabolism: Nutritional Control of Immune-Induced Growth Depression," M.E. Cook, C.C. Miller, Y. Park and Ma Pariza, *Poultry Science* 72: 1301-1305 (1993).
41. "Feeding Conjugated Linoleic Acid to Animals Partially Overcomes Catabolic Responses Due to Endotoxin Injection," Miller, C.C., Park, Y., Pariza, M, and Cook, M. Feb. 15, 1994, *Biochemical and Biophysical Research Communications,* pages 1107-1112.
42. Op. Cit. Cook, *Poultry Science,* 1993.
43. Interview with Cook.
44. Ibid.

45. Op. Cit. *Washington Post.*
46. "Obesity, Pathogenesis & Treatment, a series of reports on obesisy issues edited by G. Enzi, et. *Al,* 1981, Academic Press.
47. *William Howard Taft: The President who became Chief Justice,* by Severn, Bill 1970, David McKay company.
48. "Conjugated Linoleic Acid Reduces Body Fat," abstract only of a speech given at Environmental Biology, 96. See also U.S. Patent Number 5,554,646, dated Sep. 10, 1996.
49. Interveiw with Cook.
50. Information of Dr. Parizi provided to PharmaNutrients, Inc.
51. Interview with Cook.
52. Op. Cit. Parodi.
53. *Obesity & Weight Control: The Health Professional's Guide to Understanding & Treatment.* Edited by Frankle, R. T. 1988.
54. Ibid.
55. Op. Cit. *The Washington Post.*
56. Interview with Pariza.
57. Pariza in information to Pharmnutrients, Inc., indicates a Dr. Reid studied content in 1963 of milk fat.
58. Op Cit. Parodi.
59. Bill Phillips, *Supplement Review,* 3rd Edition.
60. Interview with Pariza.
61. Interview with Cook.
62. Interviews with Cook, Pariza.
63. Research conducted by Medstat Research Ltd., Lillestrom, Norway for the Herbal Marketing Group, HMG, Ltd., Oslo, Norway. "A pilot study with the aim of stydying the efficacy and tolerability of CLA (Tonalin) on the body composition in humans.) by Erling Thom Ph.D., Medstate Research Ltd., Liilestrom, Norway, July 1997.